REVISE BTEC TECH AWARD
Health and Social Care (2022)

PRACTICE ASSESSMENTS Plus⁺

Series Consultant: Harry Smith

Author: Elizabeth Haworth

A note from the publisher

While the publishers have made every attempt to ensure that advice on the qualification and its assessment is accurate, the official specification and associated assessment guidance materials are the only authoritative source of information and should always be referred to for definitive guidance.

This qualification is reviewed on a regular basis and may be updated in the future.

Any such updates that affect the content of this Practice Assessments Plus will be outlined at

www.pearsonfe.co.uk/BTECchanges.

For the full range of Pearson revision titles across KS2, KS3, GCSE, Functional Skills, AS/A Level and BTEC visit:
www.pearsonschools.co.uk/revise

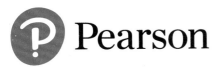

Published by Pearson Education Limited, 80 Strand, London, WC2R 0RL.

www.pearsonschoolsandfecolleges.co.uk

Copies of official specifications for all Pearson qualifications may be found on the website: qualifications.pearson.com

Text and illustrations © Pearson Education Ltd 2022

Typeset, produced and illustrated by PDQ Media

Cover illustration by © Simple Line/Shutterstock

The right of Elizabeth Haworth to be identified as author of this work has been asserted by her in accordance with the Copyright, Designs and Patents Act 1988.

First published 2022

25 24 23

10 9 8 7 6 5 4 3 2

British Library Cataloguing in Publication Data

A catalogue record for this book is available from the British Library

ISBN 978 1 292 43627 2

Copyright notice

All rights reserved. No part of this publication may be reproduced in any form or by any means (including photocopying or storing it in any medium by electronic means and whether or not transiently or incidentally to some other use of this publication) without the written permission of the copyright owner, except in accordance with the provisions of the Copyright, Designs and Patents Act 1988 or under the terms of a licence issued by the Copyright Licensing Agency, 5th Floor, Shackleton House, Hay's Galleria, 4 Battle Bridge Lane, London SE1 2HX (www.cla.co.uk). Applications for the copyright owner's written permission should be addressed to the publisher.

Printed in Slovakia by Neografia

Notes from the publisher

1. While the publishers have made every attempt to ensure that advice on the qualification and its assessment is accurate, the official specification and associated assessment guidance materials are the only authoritative source of information and should always be referred to for definitive guidance. Pearson examiners have not contributed to any sections in this resource relevant to examination papers for which they have responsibility.

2. Pearson has robust editorial processes, including answer and fact checks, to ensure the accuracy of the content in this publication, and every effort is made to ensure that this publication is free of errors. We are, however, only human, and occasionally errors do occur. Pearson is not liable for any misunderstandings that arise as a result of errors in this publication, but it is our priority to ensure that the content is accurate. If you spot an error, please do contact us at resourcescorrections@pearson.com so we can make sure that it is corrected.

Websites

Pearson Education Limited is not responsible for the content of any external internet sites. It is essential for tutors to preview each website before using it in class so as to ensure that the URL is still accurate, relevant and appropriate. We suggest that tutors bookmark useful websites and consider enabling learners to access them through the school/college intranet.

Introduction

This book has been designed to help you to practise the skills you may need for the external assessment of BTEC Tech Award **Health and Social Care**, Component 3: Health and wellbeing.

About the practice assessments

The book contains four practice assessments for the component. Unlike your actual assessment, the questions have targeted hints, guidance and support in the margin to help you understand how to tackle them:

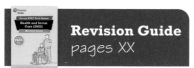 links to relevant pages in the Pearson Revise BTEC Tech Award Health and Social Care Revision Guide so you can revise the essential content. This will also help you to understand how the essential content is applied to different contexts when assessed.

 to get you started and remind you of the skills or knowledge you need to apply.

 to help you on how to approach a question, such as making a brief plan.

 to provide content that you need to learn, such as a definition or principles related to health and social care.

 to help you avoid common pitfalls.

 to remind you of content related to the question to aid your revision on that topic.

 for use with the final practice assessment to help you become familiar with answering in a given time and ways to think about allocating time for different questions.

There is space for you to write your answers to the questions within this book. However, if you require more space to complete your answers, you may want to use separate paper.

There is also an answer section at the back of the book, so you can check your answers for each practice assessment.

Check the Pearson website

For overarching guidance on the official assessment outcomes and key terms used in your assessment, please refer to the specification on the Pearson website. Check also whether you must have a calculator in your assessment.

The practice questions, support and answers in this book are provided to help you to revise the essential content in the specification, along with ways of applying your skills. Details of your actual assessment may change, so always make sure you are up to date on its format and requirements by asking your tutor or checking the Pearson website for the most up-to-date Sample Assessment Material, Mark Schemes and any past papers.

Contents

A small bit of small print

Pearson publishes Sample Assessment Material and the specification on its website. This is the official content and this book should be used in conjunction with it. The questions have been written to help you test your knowledge and skills. Remember: the real assessment may not look like this.

Practice assessment 1

Answer ALL questions.
Write your answers in the spaces provided.

Some questions must be answered with a cross in a box ☒. If you change your mind about an answer, put a line through the box ☒ and then mark your new answer with a cross ☒.

1 Identify **one** physical factor that can affect health and wellbeing.

☐ **A** Religion

☐ **B** Discrimination

☐ **C** Exercise

☐ **D** Friendship

Total for Question 1 = 1 mark

2 State **two** negative effects of smoking on health and wellbeing.

1 ....

....

2 ....

....

Total for Question 2 = 2 marks

3 State **one** environmental factor that can have an effect on health and wellbeing.

....

....

Total for Question 3 = 1 mark

Revision Guide
pages 1, 9 and 16–18

Hint

Question 1 is a multiple-choice question. This means you need to read the options carefully and discount any answers you know to be wrong. Then pick the best one from those you have left.

Hint

Negative effects are those that make a person's health and wellbeing worse **not** better.

Watch out!

In Question 2 you are being asked to state two **negative** effects. You will not get any marks for stating positive effects.

Hint

The command word **state** asks you to recall, and write down clearly, a piece of information. You do not need to explain your answer. You will not get any more marks for giving more detail.

Revision Guide
pages 13, 14
and 15.

LEARN IT!

Cultural factors relate to the characteristics of a **particular group of people**, such as their values, customs, beliefs, social habits and behaviours.

Hint

Both Questions 5 and 6 are **explain** questions. You need to recall information to identify a point then give a reason for how or why this is relevant to the question.

Hint

In Question 5 you need to identify one financial factor that will have a positive effect on health and wellbeing then give a reason why you think this is.

Watch out!

Question 6 asks you to explain **two** negative effects, so make sure you identify two factors and then give a reason for each one.

---

4 Identify **two** cultural factors that can affect health and wellbeing.

◻ **A** Religion

◻ **B** Noise pollution

◻ **C** Alcohol

◻ **D** Obesity

◻ **E** Sexual orientation

Total for Question 4 = 2 marks

5 Explain **one** positive effect of having a good income on health and wellbeing.

....

....

....

....

Total for Question 5 = 2 marks

6 Explain **two** negative effects that discrimination can have on health and wellbeing.

1 ....

....

....

....

2 ....

....

....

....

Total for Question 6 = 4 marks

7 Give **one** positive effect of supportive family relationships on the physical wellbeing of an individual.

....

....

Total for Question 7 = 1 mark

8 Explain **two** negative effects redundancy could have on the intellectual wellbeing of an individual.

1 ....

....

....

....

2 ....

....

....

....

Total for Question 8 = 4 marks

9 State **one** negative emotional effect of puberty on an individual.

....

....

Total for Question 9 = 1 mark

Revision Guide pages 12, 19 and 20.

Hint

The command word **give** means you simply need to provide the number of pieces of information asked for, with no explanation required.

Watch out!

In Question 7 you are asked to give one positive effect. Writing about more than one will not gain you extra marks and will take time you could use later on a longer question.

LEARN IT!

Redundancy means a person losing their job due to their role being deemed surplus to requirements.

Prepare

You could highlight the key words in a question to help you answer it properly. In Question 8 the key words are: two, negative, redundancy and intellectual. In Question 9 they are: one, negative, emotional and puberty.

Revision Guide
pages 13, 20
and 24.

Hint

Question 10 doesn't
mention the words positive
or negative so you can
give two positive effects,
two negative effects or
one of each. However, they
must be social effects.

Hint

When you are asked for
the correct classification
you need to identify what
group someone with that
BMI range fits into.

Hint

Make sure you use the
correct terminology.
Say whether the BMI given
is for an individual who
is underweight, healthy
weight, overweight, obese
or severely obese. Don't
use informal terms such as
'skinny' or 'fat'.

Prepare

When revising for your
assessment, make sure
you learn the correct data
for the normal ranges for
resting heart rate, blood
pressure and BMI, as well
as those considered to
be abnormal readings.

10 Explain **two** effects retirement could have on the social wellbeing
of an individual.

1 ....

....

....

....

2 ....

....

....

....

Total for Question 10 = 4 marks

11 State the correct classification for a Body Mass Index (BMI)
of 20.5 kg/m^2.

....

....

Total for Question 11 = 1 mark

Suzie's GP has informed her that her resting heart rate is too high.

12 Explain **two** potential long-term risks of having a high resting heart rate on Suzie's physical health.

1 ....

....

....

....

2 ....

....

....

....

Total for Question 12 = 4 marks

Suzie drinks more than the recommended weekly alcohol limit every weekend.

13 Explain how binge drinking will cause an increase in her resting heart rate.

....

....

....

....

Total for Question 13 = 2 marks

14 Identify **one** benefit of the person-centred approach when providing treatment for Suzie.

☐ **A** It stops her making any complaints about her treatment.

☐ **B** It saves money for health and social care services.

☐ **C** It ensures her needs are met.

☐ **D** It improves job satisfaction for health and social care workers.

Total for Question 14 = 1 mark

Revision Guide pages 10, 22 and 29.

Hint

In Question 12 make sure you identify two potential long-term risks of having a high heart rate (pulse). Then, for each one, give a reason why it is a risk to Suzie's physical health.

Hint

If you don't know the answer to a question, try to work it out using what you do know. In Question 13 think about the effects of drinking alcohol on blood pressure and how that will affect the heart.

LEARN IT!

Resting heart rate (pulse) is how fast the heart beats when a person has been still for 5 minutes. It is measured in beats per minute (bpm).

LEARN IT!

A person-centred approach puts the **individual** at the centre of health care planning.

Revision Guide
pages 20, 33,
40–45 and 50.

Hint

The command word **discuss** means you need to identify different aspects of Suzie's lifestyle that might prevent her exercising as much as she should. For each one, explain clearly why you think this.

Watch out!

Only refer to facts you have been given. Do not invent other factors or make any assumptions about Suzie.

Watch out!

Check how many marks are awarded for this question. Be sure to give enough detail to earn them all.

Prepare

When answering longer questions you need to make a point, explain your point and then add more details to justify both the point and explanation. Then repeat this with each new point you make.

The GP asks Suzie questions about her lifestyle to help them suggest ways to improve her health and wellbeing. Suzie is 25 years old, a teacher and lives with her partner. She drives the 3 km to school every day and, most evenings, she brings home planning or marking. She quickly gets out of breath when she exerts herself.

The GP advises Suzie to exercise every day and asks the practice nurse to give her some physical activity guidelines.

15 Discuss how Suzie's circumstances could affect her ability to exercise every day.

....

....

....

....

....

....

....

....

....

....

....

Total for Question 15 = 6 marks

Chen is 37 years old. He is currently unemployed, watches TV all day and eats an unhealthy diet. He also takes recreational drugs when he can afford them. He has become worried about his health and has visited his GP.

His GP says that Chen is suffering from depression and wants him to improve his health and wellbeing.

16 (a) Complete **Table 1** by:

(i) stating **three** actions his doctor could suggest that will improve Chen's health and wellbeing

(ii) giving **three** ways these actions could improve Chen's health and wellbeing.

6 marks

Three actions	Ways the actions could improve Chen's health and wellbeing
1	
2	
3	

Table 1

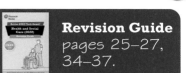

Revision Guide
pages 25–27, 34–37.

Watch out!

Don't choose actions that are too similar. If you pick one about eating, make sure the other two cover different factors.

Hint

Treat this **complete** activity like an explain question. State an action in the first column then explain why it will help Chen's health and wellbeing in the second column.

Revision Guide
pages 25–27,
34–37.

Hint

Write about both the
sources of support that
Chen's GP offers him.
Think about what the
prescription from the GP
might be for. Think about
the sort of issues that a
support group could help
Chen with.

LEARN IT!

Formal support is provided
by professionals, trained
volunteers, support groups
and charities.

Chen's GP gives him a prescription and some leaflets about local support groups.

(b) Explain **two** ways formal support could help Chen improve his health and wellbeing.

4 marks

1 ....

....

....

....

2 ....

....

....

....

Total for Question 16 = 10 marks

Dave works in sales and drives long distances to visit clients. He had a serious car accident resulting in a badly broken arm and cracked ribs. After 6 months recovering, he can now drive a car adapted to allow for the limited movement in his arm. He is now back at work as he needs the money, but he still needs to see an occupational health therapist at the hospital about his arm and his doctor for medication.

17 (a) Explain **two** possible barriers to improving Dave's health and wellbeing.

4 marks

1 ....

....

....

....

2 ....

....

....

....

Dave often meets potential clients in hotel bars and restaurants in the evenings, so he regularly eats out. During the day, he meets other customers and completes paperwork. This means he has very little free time during the week so is becoming unfit. His GP wants Dave to improve his health and wellbeing.

(b) Explain **two** obstacles that could prevent Dave improving his health and wellbeing.

4 marks

1 ....

....

....

....

2 ....

....

....

....

Total for Question 17 = 8 marks

Revision Guide
pages 19,
39–45.

LEARN IT!

A **barrier** is something unique to the health and social care system that prevents a person accessing a service.

LEARN IT!

An **obstacle** is something personal to a person that stops them moving forward, prevents action or makes action more difficult.

Watch out!

Make sure that each point you make is different. You won't be rewarded twice for making the same point, even if you give different supporting details.

Hint

For each part of question 17(a) and 17(b) you need to make a relevant point then add detail to justify each of your points. Your answers must show that you have considered Dave's needs, wishes and circumstances.

Prepare

When reading the scenario about Dave, underline any key points that you can then refer to in your answers.

Revision Guide
pages 13,
40–45.

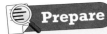

Prepare

Remember that you can draw on what you have learned throughout your whole health and social care course to help you answer this question, not just this component.

Hint

Using knowledge from the whole course, consider how Mela's partner has affected her social development from when she met them to now.

Hint

You need to write about the personal obstacles that Mela now faces, and the effects they could have on her social development.

Watch out!

Check your answer to make sure you have answered the question. Make any changes neatly and clearly. Check your writing, spelling, punctuation and grammar, to help the assessor read and understand your answer better.

Mela is 56 years old. Her partner of 35 years has recently died and she is finding it hard to adjust to being on her own. She has no family and very few friends because her partner was happy to stay at home every night rather than socialise with others. She is lonely and often comfort eats, so has put weight on. Mela decides she needs to lose weight and meet new people.

18 Discuss how Mela's circumstances may affect her social development as she tries to achieve her goals.

....

....

....

....

....

....

....

....

....

....

....

....

Total for Question 18 = 6 marks

TOTAL FOR PAPER = 60 MARKS

Practice assessment 2

Answer ALL questions.
Write your answers in the spaces provided.

Some questions must be answered with a cross in a box ☒. If you change your mind about an answer, put a line through the box ☒ and then mark your new answer with a cross ☒.

Revision Guide
pages 8, 14
and 15.

1 Identify **one** economic factor that can affect health and wellbeing.

☐ **A** Bullying

☐ **B** Stress

☐ **C** Pollution

☐ **D** Savings

Total for Question 1 = 1 mark

Watch out!

Question 1 asks you to identify an economic factor. Money can cause stress, but that doesn't mean that stress is an economic factor.

Hint

The word **identify** used in a multiple-choice question means you need to pick the correct answer from the choices offered. Eliminate the ones you know are wrong then, if you are still unsure, choose the most likely remaining option.

2 State **two** positive effects of regular exercise on health and wellbeing.

1 ....

....

2 ....

....

Total for Question 2 = 2 marks

Watch out!

In Question 2 you are being asked to state two positive effects of regular exercise. You will not get any marks if you write about any factor other than exercise.

3 State **one** cultural factor that can have an effect on health and wellbeing.

....

....

Total for Question 3 = 1 mark

Hint

When you are asked to **state** a factor or an effect, be clear and concise. Simply give the fact asked for.

Revision Guide
pages 13, 18, 25–28.

Watch out!

Look carefully at the number of options you are asked to identify in a multiple-choice question. Here you need to identify two, not just one.

Hint

In **explain** questions such as Questions 5 and 6 you need to identify a point and then support your point by giving more detail to show why it is relevant to the question.

Hint

In Question 5 you need to identify one **negative** effect of social exclusion on health and wellbeing then explain why you think this. Make sure you don't give any positive effects.

LEARN IT!

Social factors relate to interactions between people, which means making connections and communicating with others.

Hint

When asked about how a factor can affect health and wellbeing, you can choose any aspects of health and wellbeing for your answer (physical, intellectual, emotional or social).

---

4 Identify **two** lifestyle factors that can affect health and wellbeing.

☐ **A** Community participation

☐ **B** Balanced diet

☐ **C** Anxiety

☐ **D** Religion

☐ **E** Physical activity

Total for Question 4 = 2 marks

5 Explain **one** negative effect of social exclusion on health and wellbeing.

....

....

....

....

Total for Question 5 = 2 marks

6 Explain **two** positive effects of a clean, safe and well-kept home environment on health and wellbeing.

1 ....

....

....

....

2 ....

....

....

....

Total for Question 6 = 4 marks

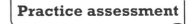

7 Give **one** negative effect of a serious illness on the emotional wellbeing of an individual.

....

....

Total for Question 7 = 1 mark

Revision Guide pages 3, 19 and 20.

Hint

In Question 7 you need to give a precise answer that uses correct terminology and language from the specification. You don't need to explain your answer.

8 Explain **two** positive effects of starting work for the first time on the social wellbeing of a young adult.

1 ....

....

....

....

2 ....

....

....

....

Total for Question 8 = 4 marks

Watch out!

Check to make sure you have answered the question. In Question 8 if you write about any life event other than starting work for the first time or any effects other than social effects, you will not gain the marks.

9 State **one** positive physical effect of the menopause on an individual.

....

....

Total for Question 9 = 1 mark

Prepare

Make sure you check the number of marks on offer for each question and answer every question. In Question 8 you have to identify and explain two different positive effects.

LEARN IT!

The **menopause** marks the end of a woman's fertility and usually occurs between the ages of 45 and 55.

Revision Guide
pages 20 and 22.

Hint

Here you need to clearly state two effects (which can be positive and/or negative) and then provide a reason for each, using a connective word to help you. Use words such as 'because' and 'therefore'.

Hint

Read the question carefully to ensure that your answer has the right focus. Question 10 asks for effects of **redundancy** on **emotional** wellbeing.

Hint

Here you need to identify what group someone with that resting heart rate fits into. Say whether their resting heart rate is lower than normal, normal or higher than normal.

Prepare

Remember, you need to learn the normal ranges for resting heart rate, blood pressure and Body Mass Index (BMI).

---

10 Explain **two** effects redundancy could have on the emotional wellbeing of an individual.

1 ....

....

....

....

2 ....

....

....

....

Total for Question 10 = 4 marks

11 State the correct classification for a resting heart rate of below 60 bpm.

....

....

Total for Question 11 = 1 mark

> Muhammad is 65 and needs an operation to replace his knee, but his consultant tells him that his BMI is too high.

12 Explain **two** potential short-term risks of having a high BMI on Muhammad's physical health.

1 ....

....

....

....

2 ....

....

....

....

Total for Question 12 = 4 marks

> Muhammad sits at a desk working on a computer all day at work.

13 Explain how a lack of exercise may cause an increase in Muhammad's BMI.

....

....

....

....

Total for Question 13 = 2 marks

14 Identify **one** way in which a person-centred approach takes into account the person's circumstances.

☐ **A** It includes days off for the care worker.

☐ **B** It includes the person's age and ability.

☐ **C** It doesn't include the person's living conditions.

☐ **D** It includes where the care worker lives.

Total for Question 14 = 1 mark

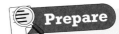

Revision Guide
pages 8, 21, 24 and 29.

LEARN IT!

BMI stands for **Body Mass Index** and is a measure of the amount of fat in a person's body.

Prepare

You need to learn the short- and long-term risks to an individual of having abnormal health indicators, such as resting heart rate, blood pressure and BMI.

Hint

Question 12 expects you to give two distinct answers, as indicated by the numbering.

Hint

Think about what doesn't happen to the food a person eats if they do not move all day? What might happen if they do this day after day?

LEARN IT!

A person's circumstances are the things that directly affect the person in the situation they find themselves in.

Revision Guide
pages 7, 25, 34 and 40.

Hint

For this **discuss** question you need to identify different aspects of Muhammad's lifestyle that might help him to eat more healthily and/or prevent him from doing so. Make sure you support each of the points you make with a clear explanation.

Watch out!

Your answer must be relevant to Muhammad's lifestyle and consider the points given in the scenario. Highlight the key points before you start, to help you stay focused.

Watch out!

The space allocated should be more than enough to complete your answer.

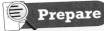 **Prepare**

This is a longer question worth 6 marks. You need to make sure that each of your points is well developed. Include a range of different aspects and how they relate to each other.

The practice nurse asks Muhammad questions about his lifestyle so she can suggest ways to improve his health and wellbeing. Muhammad is an accountant and lives with his wife in a house in the country. They have lots of friends and eat out most weekends. He and his work colleagues go out for lunch every day.

The practice nurse suggests that Muhammad eat a healthy diet.

15 Discuss how Muhammad's circumstances could affect his ability to eat a healthy diet.

....

....

....

....

....

....

....

....

....

....

....

Total for Question 15 = 6 marks

Leanne is a self-employed website developer. She works long hours in her home office and often at weekends too. She gets so engrossed in what she's doing that she often forgets to eat or just grabs a snack. Leanne is underweight and has difficulty sleeping at night, no matter how tired she is when she goes to bed.

She visits her GP who wants to help Leanne improve her health and wellbeing.

16 (a) Complete **Table 1** by:

(i) stating **three** actions her doctor could suggest to improve Leanne's health and wellbeing

(ii) giving **three** ways these actions could improve Leanne's health and wellbeing.

6 marks

Three actions	Ways the actions could improve Leanne's health and wellbeing
1	
2	
3	

Table 1

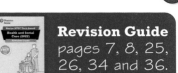

Revision Guide
pages 7, 8, 25, 26, 34 and 36.

Watch out!

Make sure you choose actions that are different so that they don't have the same explanation.

Hint

Give a point in the first column and then justify it in the second column by explaining how the action will help Leanne.

Revision Guide
pages 7, 8, 25, 26, 34 and 38.

Hint

In Question 16(b) make sure you only refer to the sources of informal support identified in the question. Don't invent other sources of support for Leanne.

LEARN IT!

Informal support is provided by people who are not paid or trained to do so. They do it because they want to help.

Leanne lives with her husband. She has two sisters who live nearby and a best friend who lives a few miles away. She speaks to her best friend and her sisters on the phone most weeks.

(b) Explain **two** ways informal support could help Leanne improve her health and wellbeing.

`4 marks`

1 ....

....

....

....

2 ....

....

....

....

Total for Question 16 = 10 marks

Revision Guide
pages 14, 20,
39–43 and 45.

Abena has recently arrived in the UK to start a new job. She plans to live with her cousin. She collapses at the airport and is rushed to hospital with a very high temperature. She is put in an isolation ward on her own while the doctors try to work out what is wrong with her. She speaks very little English and feels unwell.

17 (a) Explain **two** possible barriers to improving Abena's health and wellbeing.

4 marks

1 ....
....
....
....

2 ....
....
....
....

Hint

You need to identify barriers in 17(a) and obstacles in 17(b). Make sure you read the scenarios provided very carefully to make sure you identify those that are relevant to Abena.

Watch out!

Check your answer. If you have written about obstacles instead of barriers, and vice versa, you will not gain any marks.

Abena is well enough to be discharged from hospital. Her cousin doesn't drive and lives in a small village 15 miles away. She asks a friend to drive her to collect Abena. Abena still needs to attend follow-up appointments for more tests at the hospital, but she has no money as she hasn't been able to start her new job yet. The only bus passes the hospital twice a day.

(b) Explain **two** obstacles that could prevent Abena from improving her health and wellbeing.

4 marks

1 ....
....
....
....

2 ....
....
....
....

Hint

Once you have identified the barriers and obstacles you need to clearly explain why each of these may stop Abena accessing the services she needs to improve her health and wellbeing.

Prepare

When reading the information given, highlight key points to help focus your answer. Remember, your answers must show that you have considered Abena's needs, wishes and circumstances.

Total for Question 17 = 8 marks

Hint

This is a longer question worth 6 marks. For each point you make explain your point and add more detail to justify both the point and explanation.

Hint

You need to write about the specific personal obstacles that James faces and the effects these could have on his emotional development.

Hint

Think about what you have learned about sensory impairment and ill health, and their impacts on health and wellbeing. Relate your learning to the possible effects on James's emotional development.

Watch out!

Don't assume that James's circumstances will only affect him negatively. Remember that a balance of positive and negative effects gives a more rounded answer and shows your knowledge and understanding of the topic.

James is 18 years old and deaf. He also has a medical condition, which isn't serious but means he has missed quite a lot of school due to being ill or attending medical appointments. His parents are determined to help him and always do everything they can to support him. He is about to begin college.

18 Discuss how James's circumstances may affect his emotional development in early adulthood.

....

....

....

....

....

....

....

....

....

....

....

Total for Question 18 = 6 marks

TOTAL FOR PAPER = 60 MARKS

Practice assessment 3

Answer ALL questions.
Write your answers in the spaces provided.

Some questions must be answered with a cross in a box ☒. If you change your mind about an answer, put a line through the box ☒ and then mark your new answer with a cross ☒.

1 Identify **one** lifestyle factor that can affect health and wellbeing.

☐ **A** Inheritance

☐ **B** Neglect

☐ **C** Cardiovascular disease

☐ **D** Smoking

Total for Question 1 = 1 mark

2 State **two** negative effects of an unhealthy diet on health and wellbeing.

1 ....

....

2 ....

....

Total for Question 2 = 2 marks

3 State **one** economic factor that can have an effect on health and wellbeing.

....

....

Total for Question 3 = 1 mark

Revision Guide
pages 7, 15, 25–28.

Watch out!

Question 1 asks you to identify a **lifestyle factor**. A lifestyle factor is a choice people make about how they live. Don't confuse this with physical, social, cultural, economic or environmental factors.

Hint

The word **identify** means you need to pick the number of correct answers that the question asks for from the choices offered. In this question you need to pick one.

Hint

In Question 2 you need to provide two negative effects of an unhealthy diet on any aspects of a person's physical, intellectual, emotional or social wellbeing.

Hint

The command word **state** means you need to give a precise answer that uses the correct terminology. There is no need to add any extra detail.

Revision Guide
pages 1, 11
and 14.

Watch out!

In this multiple-choice question, some answers might seem as though they are physical factors but are actually social or emotional factors, so think carefully about the answers you pick.

LEARN IT!

Religion is a **cultural factor** in a person's health and wellbeing. People who belong to the same religion share certain beliefs, values, behaviours, customs and social norms.

Hint

Question 5 is an **explain** question so you need to identify one positive effect and give one reason to support your point, rather than write a list of positive effects.

Hint

For Question 6 you can write about substance abuse in general or identify a specific substance. Remember to explain how the substance affects a person negatively. The effects can be physical, intellectual, emotional or social.

4 Identify **two** physical factors that can affect health and wellbeing.

- ☐ **A** Supportive relationships
- ☐ **B** Regular exercise
- ☐ **C** Substance misuse
- ☐ **D** Bullying
- ☐ **E** Culture

Total for Question 4 = 2 marks

5 Explain **one** positive effect of religion on health and wellbeing.

....

....

....

....

Total for Question 5 = 2 marks

6 Explain **two** negative effects of substance abuse on health and wellbeing.

1 ....

....

....

....

2 ....

....

....

....

Total for Question 6 = 4 marks

7 Give **one** positive effect of a serious illness on the emotional wellbeing of an individual.

....

....

Total for Question 7 = 1 mark

8 Explain **two** negative effects of bereavement on the physical wellbeing of an individual.

1 ....

....

....

....

2 ....

....

....

....

Total for Question 8 = 4 marks

9 State **one** negative social effect of a life-changing accident on an individual.

....

....

Total for Question 9 = 1 mark

Revision Guide
pages 3, 4, 13 and 19.

Hint

The command word **give** means you only need to state one effect. You need to be clear and concise.

Hint

In **explain** questions such as Question 8, use connecting words such as 'because' and 'therefore' to help you link your ideas and develop your point.

Watch out!

Check to make sure you have answered the question. In Question 8 the life event is bereavement and the type of wellbeing is physical, so make sure those are what you write about.

LEARN IT!

A life-changing accident is one where the individual is left with permanent changes to their body, such as scars, loss of a limb or sight, or a brain injury.

Revision Guide
pages 1, 4, 19, 20 and 23.

Hint

Underline or highlight the key points in the question, to make sure you focus your answer correctly. Here the key points are **divorce** and **intellectual wellbeing**. The effects you give could be positive or negative.

Hint

Question 10 is an **explain** question so, as well as identifying two effects, you also need to say how each one could affect a person's intellectual wellbeing.

Watch out!

You need to give two **different** answers for each part of Question 10. You can't just give two details about the same effect.

Prepare

Blood pressure is an important indicator of health. Learn the normal range and also make sure you know the effects of high or low blood pressure on the body.

---

10 Explain **two** effects divorce could have on the intellectual wellbeing of an individual.

1 ....

....

....

....

2 ....

....

....

....

Total for Question 10 = 4 marks

11 State the correct classification for a blood pressure of 150/97 mmHg.

....

....

Total for Question 11 = 1 mark

Delphine's doctor says that her heart rate (pulse) recovery from exercise is too slow – it takes too long for her heart rate to return to normal.

12 Explain **two** potential risks to Delphine's health of having slow heart rate (pulse) recovery from exercise.

1 ....

....

....

....

2 ....

....

....

....

Total for Question 12 = 4 marks

Delphine smokes to relax.

13 Explain how smoking will cause an increase in the time it takes for Delphine's heart rate (pulse) to return to normal after exercise.

....

....

....

....

Total for Question 13 = 2 marks

14 Identify **one** feature of a person-centred approach.

☐ **A** A partnership between the individual and the health professionals

☐ **B** Treatment remains the same regardless of the circumstances of the individual

☐ **C** The individual is given an exercise plan to follow for 6 months

☐ **D** Costs are kept as low as possible for the services involved

Total for Question 14 = 1 mark

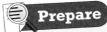

Revision Guide
pages 9, 22 and 29.

🔍 **Prepare**

If a person's heart takes longer than normal to return to normal after exercise this shows that they are unfit. You need to learn what this might mean for that person's long-term health.

Hint

Question 13 is an **explain** question so don't forget to make a point then add detail to justify why you have made that point.

Hint

When answering Question 14 read the definition of a person-centred approach given in the LEARN IT box and decide which feature supports that definition.

LEARN IT!

The person-centred approach puts the individual at the heart of health care planning and takes into account an individual's needs (to reduce health risks), wishes and circumstances.

Revision Guide
pages 9, 27
and 40–45

Hint

The command word is **discuss**, so you need to identify and explain. Refer to all the information in the scenario to identify the most relevant factors likely to prevent Daphne from stopping smoking.

Watch out!

Remember that the assessor needs to be able to read and understand your answer so write neatly and take care with your spelling, punctuation and grammar.

Watch out!

The space allocated is a guide as to how much you need to write to answer the question fully if you write neatly on the lines provided.

Prepare

When answering longer questions, try to structure your answer so it displays your knowledge and understanding in a well-developed and logical discussion.

Delphine is experiencing breathlessness and pains in her chest so she visits her GP. She is 32 years old, runs her own online business from home and lives on her own. She smokes to relax, loves to party and often goes out drinking with her friends. Her friends all smoke.

The GP suggests that Delphine stops smoking.

15 Discuss how Delphine's circumstances could affect her ability to stop smoking.

....

....

....

....

....

....

....

....

....

....

....

Total for Question 15 = 6 marks

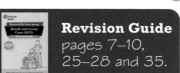

Revision Guide
pages 7–10,
25–28 and 35.

Eamonn is 57 years old and works long hours, standing up all day. He and his colleagues frequently go outside for a smoking break during the day. After their shift they go to the pub for a few pints and often pick up a takeaway meal on the way home.

He visits his GP for his annual check-up. The GP wants Eamonn to improve his health and wellbeing.

16 (a) Complete **Table 1** by:

(i) stating **three** actions his doctor could suggest to improve Eamonn's health and wellbeing

(ii) giving **three** ways these actions could improve Eamonn's health and wellbeing.

6 marks

Three actions	Ways the actions could improve Eamonn's health and wellbeing
1	
2	
3	

Table 1

Watch out!

Remember that the actions must be based on three **different** lifestyle factors. That way you won't write about the same one twice by mistake and lose marks.

Hint

Justify each action in the second column by explaining how it will help Eamonn if he does as the doctor suggests.

Revision Guide
pages 19, 25–
28, 35–37.

Hint

In Question 16(b) think about what formal sources of support Eamonn could access to help him with his dependence on alcohol and smoking.

Watch out!

Only write about formal support. If you write about informal support, you won't get any marks, even if you correctly identify sources of informal support. Always make sure you answer the question asked.

Eamonn has lived on his own since his wife died 3 years ago.
He is dependent on alcohol and cigarettes.

(b) Explain **two** ways formal support could help Eamonn improve his health and wellbeing.

4 marks

1 ....

....

....

....

2 ....

....

....

....

Total for Question 16 = 10 marks

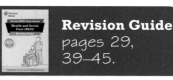

Revision Guide
pages 29,
39–45.

Rosie is 7 years old and lives with her dad in a tower block. She has asthma. The flat is damp, which makes her asthma worse. Dad works for minimum wage in the local supermarket. Rosie needs to attend the local hospital for breathing exercises every week and to see the practice nurse to review her asthma medication. The hospital and surgery are at the top of a steep hill about a mile away and it takes two bus journeys to get there.

17 (a) Explain **two** possible barriers to improving Rosie's health and wellbeing.

4 marks

1 ....

....

....

....

2 ....

....

....

....

Rosie's dad is made redundant and he is too embarrassed to ask for help. He feels he is letting Rosie down, as he doesn't want to leave the flat. Rosie's regular hospital appointment is on Friday afternoon.

(b) Explain **two** obstacles that could prevent Rosie from accessing the services she needs to improve her health and wellbeing.

4 marks

1 ....

....

....

....

2 ....

....

....

....

Total for Question 17 = 8 marks

LEARN IT!

A **barrier** is something about the health and social care system itself. An **obstacle** is something particular to the person that prevents them accessing a service.

LEARN IT!

Remember the different types of barriers and obstacles. **Barriers** can be physical, social, cultural, sensory, language, geographical, resources or financial. **Obstacles** can be emotional/psychological, time constraints, availability of resources, unachievable targets or lack of support.

Hint

Always look for the words in bold. In both parts of this question **two** is in bold. Make sure your answers only mention **two** barriers in 17(a) and **two** obstacles in 17(b).

Prepare

Read both parts of the question carefully as this will provide you with the information you need. Your answers must show that you have considered Rosie's specific needs, wishes and circumstances.

Revision Guide
pages 13, 40–45.

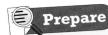 **Prepare**

Before answering the question, read the scenario carefully and highlight key points that will affect Tahira's physical development.

Hint

The command word in this question is **discuss**, so for each point you make explain it then justify it with more detail.

Hint

Think about what Tahira eats and whether she has much chance to build up her muscles, get fresh air or sleep well.

Watch out!

This question doesn't ask you to focus on positive or negative factors so you could include some of each, even if there are more of one type than the other. This gives a better answer.

Hint

Make sure your writing is neat and that you take care with spelling, grammar and punctuation.

> Tahira is 10 years old. Her mother is disabled and attends a day care centre during the day. Tahira is her mother's main carer when she is not at school. She relies on her school lunches for a proper meal and prepares basic meals such as beans on toast in the evenings for herself and her mother. She gets up early in the morning to get her mum up and to do jobs such as cleaning and washing. She is unable to join in any after-school clubs or weekend activities with her friends, as she needs to look after her mother.

18 Discuss how Tahira's circumstances may affect her physical development in childhood.

....

....

....

....

....

....

....

....

....

....

....

Total for Question 18 = 6 marks

TOTAL FOR PAPER = 60 MARKS

Practice assessment 4

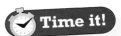

Answer ALL questions.
Write your answers in the spaces provided.

Some questions must be answered with a cross in a box ☒. If you change your mind about an answer, put a line through the box ☒ and then mark your new answer with a cross ☒.

1 Identify **one** environmental factor that can affect health and wellbeing.

☐ **A** Poor living conditions

☐ **B** Alcohol

☐ **C** Cystic fibrosis

☐ **D** Gender roles

Total for Question 1 = 1 mark

2 State **two** negative effects of substance abuse on health and wellbeing.

1 ....

....

2 ....

....

Total for Question 2 = 2 marks

3 State **one** physical factor that can have an effect on health and wellbeing.

....

....

Total for Question 3 = 1 mark

Revision Guide
pages 1–6, 11, 16 and 17.

⏱ Time it!

Time yourself completing this paper. Remember that the time allowed for your actual assessment might vary so check the front of the assessment paper and with your teacher or tutor.

Hint

Identify means that you need to select a piece of information from the list given. Here you need to pick the only correct answer from the options.

Hint

Double-check the number of options the question asks for. If you select two answers for Question 1, you will not gain the mark.

Hint

Remember that **state** means the same as 'give'. In Questions 2 and 3 you need to provide the number of accurate facts asked for in the question, making sure you use the correct terminology.

Revision Guide
pages 4, 7, 12, 13, 25 and 38.

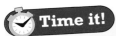

Watch out!

In this multiple-choice question you are asked for **two** correct answers, not just one. Always read the question carefully to avoid mistakes such as picking the wrong number of answers.

Time it!

Don't spend too long on short-answer questions such as Question 5. You should spend about 1 minute per mark to allow more planning time for the longer questions.

Hint

In an **explain** question there should be two parts to your response. In Question 5 you need to specify one negative effect of poor nutrition and then give a reason for your answer.

Hint

In Question 6 you won't get a mark for saying 'they'll feel supported' or 'they have support' as this is stated in the question.

4 Identify **two** social factors that can affect health and wellbeing.

- ☐ **A** Social inclusion
- ☐ **B** Smoking
- ☐ **C** Employment
- ☐ **D** Stress
- ☐ **E** Discrimination

Total for Question 4 = 2 marks

5 Explain **one** negative effect of poor nutrition on health and wellbeing.

....

....

....

....

Total for Question 5 = 2 marks

6 Explain **two** positive effects of supportive relationships on health and wellbeing.

1 ....

....

....

....

2 ....

....

....

....

Total for Question 6 = 4 marks

7 Give **one** negative effect of moving house on the intellectual wellbeing of an individual.

....

....

Total for Question 7 = 1 mark

8 Explain **two** positive effects of starting college on the emotional wellbeing of an individual.

1 ....

....

....

....

2 ....

....

....

....

Total for Question 8 = 4 marks

9 State **one** positive intellectual effect of leaving home on an individual.

....

....

Total for Question 9 = 1 mark

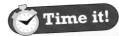

Revision Guide
pages 1, 16
and 20.

Hint

Questions with the command word **give** want you to provide a concise and accurate fact. No explanation or extra detail is needed.

Time it!

Aim to answer questions that are worth one mark in a maximum of a minute each. You can spend about 5 minutes on Question 8, which needs more detail.

Hint

In Question 8 you are being asked to think about the life event starting college and explain two of the effects of this event on **emotional** wellbeing. Imagine how you might **feel** if you were starting college.

Watch out!

Make sure you answer the question asked. In Question 9 does it ask for a positive or negative effect? Are you asked to 'state' or to 'explain' an effect? Don't overwrite!

Revision Guide
pages 1, 20, 24.

Hint

In questions where you are asked for effects, without the words positive or negative, you can give either or a mixture of both.

LEARN IT!

Try to refer to two **different** components of physical health, which could include: healthy body systems; regular exercise; a healthy diet; regular sleep patterns; access to shelter and warmth; good personal hygiene.

Hint

In Question 11 you are asked to identify what this specific BMI tells you about the weight of an individual. Use the correct terminology rather than an informal word in your answer.

Time it!

Allow yourself time to check your answers to make sure you haven't given any inaccurate facts or made careless mistakes.

---

10 Explain **two** effects that starting school could have on the physical wellbeing of a child.

1 ....

....

....

....

2 ....

....

....

....

Total for Question 10 = 4 marks

11 State the correct classification for a Body Mass Index (BMI) of 36.2 kg/m².

....

....

Total for Question 11 = 1 mark

Katie's GP has told her that her blood pressure is too low.

12 Explain **two** potential risks of having a low blood pressure for Katie's physical health.

1 ....

....

....

....

2 ....

....

....

....

Total for Question 12 = 4 marks

Katie's diet is not healthy according to the Eatwell Guide guidelines.

13 Explain how an unhealthy diet will eventually cause an increase in her blood pressure.

....

....

....

....

Total for Question 13 = 2 marks

14 Identify **one** benefit of a person-centred approach for a health and social care service.

☐ **A** The individual has more confidence in recommendations

☐ **B** Fewer complaints about health and social care services and workers

☐ **C** Increased support available for individuals

☐ **D** Improved independence for the individual

Total for Question 14 = 1 mark

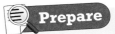

Revision Guide pages 23, 25, 29 and 32.

Prepare

If a person's blood pressure is too low it can be as serious as high blood pressure. You need to know what this might mean for that person's long-term health.

Hint

Here, you are being asked to apply what you have learned about blood pressure to the health of a particular individual, to show that you know how specific factors will affect their **physical** health.

Watch out!

Question 14 is asking how a person-centred approach helps the health and social care services or service providers not an individual.

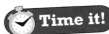 **Time it!**

Practise answering assessment questions against the clock so that you are well prepared to work under exam conditions.

Revision Guide
pages 10, 20,
28, 29, 35–38.

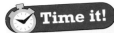

Time it!

Make a quick plan for longer answers like this one to ensure you stay focused and make the best use of your time. Leave yourself a minute or two to check over your answer.

Prepare

Carefully consider all the information that you have been given and identify which are the most important or relevant factors to Elliot's ability to drink less alcohol.

Hint

Question 15 asks you to **discuss**, so read the question at least twice before answering, to make sure you have understood all the key points you need to cover.

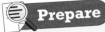

Hint

Your discussion needs to be explained logically and clearly, and show you have considered how your points interrelate. You can link them together by using connective words such as 'because' and 'so.'

Elliot lives with his husband. They are both retired but Elliot does voluntary work as a magistrate, which he intends to continue to do until the age of 70. His work as a magistrate can be demanding and very stressful and Elliot drinks alcohol every evening to relax. The couple's social life revolves around meals and drinks out.

At Elliot's annual health check the practice nurse suggests that Elliot drinks less alcohol.

15 Discuss how Elliot's circumstances could affect his ability to drink less alcohol.

....

....

....

....

....

....

....

....

....

....

....

Total for Question 15 = 6 marks

Priya was a professional dancer until she injured her knee last year. Although her weight is within the normal range, she is heavier than she used to be. She lives on pasta, cheese, broccoli and sweet foods. She drinks sugary fizzy drinks. Priya loves exercise but has stopped because of her knee.

She visits her GP for advice on how to improve her health and wellbeing.

16 (a) Complete **Table 1** by:

    (i) stating **three** actions her doctor could suggest to improve Priya's health and wellbeing

    (ii) giving **three** ways these actions could improve Priya's health and wellbeing.

6 marks

Three actions	Ways the actions could improve Priya's health and wellbeing
1	
2	
3	

Table 1

Revision Guide
pages 7, 8, 25, 26, 36–38.

Watch out!

Remember to try to pick actions based on three different lifestyle factors. The detail about food is only one possible factor for you to identify.

Watch out!

Although you are being asked to complete a table, you still need to write neatly and clearly in the spaces provided so the assessor can easily read your answers.

Revision Guide
pages 7, 8, 25, 26 and 38.

Hint

In Question 16(b) think about different ways Priya's parents and younger brother can separately help her follow the actions the doctor has suggested.

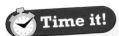 **Time it!**

Questions 16(a) and 16(b) are worth 10 marks out of a possible total of 60 for the whole assessment. Check the total number of marks in your final assessment and the number of minutes allowed, and remember to divide your time up accordingly.

Priya still lives with her parents and younger brother.

(b) Explain **two** ways informal support could help Priya improve her health and wellbeing.

4 marks

1 ....

....

....

....

2 ....

....

....

....

Total for Question 16 = 10 marks

Ivan has recently had a brain tumour successfully removed but has been told that he needs to take medication for the rest of his life, as well as regular hospital appointments to check that the tumour has not returned. He lives on his own, and he isn't allowed to return to work yet or drive for 12 months. The nearest hospital with the scanner he needs is 5 miles away in one direction and his GP is 3 miles away in the opposite direction.

17 (a) Explain **two** possible barriers to improving Ivan's health and wellbeing.

4 marks

1 ....

   ....

   ....

   ....

2 ....

   ....

   ....

   ....

Ivan constantly worries about his brain tumour returning. He sometimes drinks alcohol to reduce his anxiety, which is against the medical advice he has been given. He is also reluctant to go out with his friends as he is still scared that he will have a seizure, which used to happen regularly before his operation. As a result, he is losing touch with his friends.

(b) Explain **two** obstacles that could prevent Ivan from accessing the services he needs to improve his health and wellbeing.

4 marks

1 ....

   ....

   ....

   ....

2 ....

   ....

   ....

   ....

Total for Question 17 = 8 marks

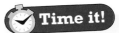

Revision Guide pages 10, 19, 29, 39–45.

⏱ **Time it!**

Check how much time you have left, as you will need to leave at least 8 minutes to answer the final question.

Hint

You should correctly identify **two** factors from the scenario that could be barriers to improving Ivan's health and wellbeing. Then expand on each factor to provide a clear explanation of why it could be a barrier.

Hint

Remember the difference between barriers and obstacles. They both make access to services difficult, but **barriers** relate to the health and social care system, whereas **obstacles** relate to an individual.

Hint

Use the additional information in part (b) to identify the obstacles. Remember, your answers must show that you have considered Ivan's needs, wishes and circumstances.

Revision Guide
pages 1 and 20

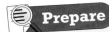

Prepare

Highlight key points in the scenario that may affect Noah's intellectual development in childhood.

Watch out!

Make sure you focus on Noah's intellectual development and don't write about his physical, social or cultural development.

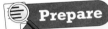

Prepare

Remember to revise your knowledge from other components of your course. You will need to draw on what you have learned about intellectual development in early childhood here.

Time it!

Make sure you leave at least 5 minutes at the end of your assessment to check that you are happy with your answers. Make any necessary changes neatly, clearly crossing out any wrong answers.

Time it!

Review how long it took to complete your assessment. Think about whether you could have allocated your time differently to improve your performance.

> Noah is 7 years old. His mum hated school so never bothers listening to him read or telling him things that will increase his general knowledge. She prefers to spend her time on her phone. If she thinks it's too cold or wet to go out, she sometimes tells school he is unwell and doesn't take him, although Noah is bored at home. His dad works long shifts and Noah is usually getting ready for bed by the time he gets home.

18 Discuss how Noah's circumstances may affect his intellectual development in childhood.

....

....

....

....

....

....

....

....

....

....

....

Total for Question 18 = 6 marks

TOTAL FOR PAPER = 60 MARKS

Answers

Use this section to check your answers.
- For questions with clear correct answers, these are provided.
- For questions where individuals may give the correct answer phrased in different ways or there may be more than one correct answer, this is noted along with example answers.
- For questions that require longer answers, bullet points are provided to indicate key points you could include in your answer or how your answer could be structured. **Your answer should be written using sentences and paragraphs** and might include some of these points but not necessarily all of them.

> The questions and sample answers are provided to help you revise content and skills. Ask your tutor or check the Pearson website for the most up-to-date Sample Assessment Material, past papers and mark schemes to get an indication of the actual assessment and what this requires of you. Details of the actual assessment may change so always make sure you are up to date.

Practice assessment 1

(pages 1–10)

1 C

2 Answers could include any **two** from:
- increased blood pressure/risk of heart attack/stroke
- increased risk of gum disease
- increased risk of bronchitis/emphysema/asthma
- increased risk of cancer/thrombosis
- increased risk of smoker's cough
- Poorer self-esteem due to:
  o wrinkled face
  o stained hands and nails
  o smell on breath and clothes
- poor self-concept if unable to quit
- social exclusion due to having to smoke outside.

3 Answers could include any **one** from:
- air pollution
- noise pollution
- light pollution
- housing needs
- housing conditions
- housing location
- home environment
- sanitation/waste disposal
- water quality/pollution
- extreme weather and climate change
- geographical risk factors (earthquakes, flooding etc)
- presence of pests and disease carriers
- population density.

4 A and E

5 Answers can include any **one** from:

the ability to:
- more easily afford a greater variety of foods or outsource cooking/delivery to create a more balanced diet; improving physical wellbeing
- afford more leisure services, luxuries, holidays, hobbies and social activities; improving social and emotional wellbeing
- afford better housing in cleaner/safer/greener environments; improving physical wellbeing
- feel financially secure; improving emotional wellbeing
- afford a greater array of learning opportunities/educational resources; improving intellectual wellbeing.

6 Answers could include any **two** from:
- social isolation; making the person feel lonely
- social isolation; leading to poorer grades if the student doesn't attend school as a result of discrimination
- low self-esteem; due to being made to feel different
- anxiety; due to feeling judged by people
- stress; due to worrying about what people think of them
- increased blood pressure; caused by stress
- insomnia; caused by anxiety
- distress; caused by being treated with a lack of respect
- anger; at being treated differently
- lack of concentration; due to being distracted by feeling upset
- unhappiness; due to being treated unfairly
- driven to alcohol, smoking or substance abuse; to forget how being treated
- poorer life opportunities; less likely to access higher education if feeling unable to attend for fear of being discriminated against
- financial impact; not being considered for jobs or for promotion.

7 Answers could include any **one** from:
- more active
- healthier diet
- healthier relationship with alcohol/stimulants
- better sleeping habits
- better support to recover during illness/injury.

8 Answers could include any **two** from:
- worried/anxious/stressed; so less able to concentrate
- less money available; so less able to afford to travel and learn about new cultures
- less money available; so less able to afford learning opportunities, such as courses, subscriptions and books.

9 Answers could include any **one** from:
- mood swings/moodiness
- anxiety or depression
- unhappy/self-conscious/embarrassed/worried about skin, changing shape or other physical effects of puberty.

10 Answers could include any **two** from:
- increased social interaction; because of more time to spend with friends/family
- make new friends; as more opportunities to join new groups/take up new hobbies/travel
- able to contribute to conversation/improved social skills; as more able to keep up with the news/learn new things
- improved relationships; as more relaxed and less stressed with work
- reduced social interaction; because no longer socialising with colleagues/clients/attending work-related events
- lower income; less income as may be relying on a pension
- depression/boredom due to losing position/purpose in life.

11 Healthy weight/normal weight/ideal weight

12 Answers could include any **two** from:
- higher blood pressure; because the heart is working harder to push her blood round her body
- increased risks of heart attack/stroke; because the heart is working harder, requiring more oxygen than the body can provide, resulting in cell death over time
- increased risk of death; because the heart is having to work harder over a given period of time.

13 Drinking too much alcohol causes blood pressure to increase; so the heart is having to beat faster/work harder to push blood around the body, leading to a higher heart rate.

Also acceptable:

Alcohol may affect the balance of the nervous system, causing the heart to beat faster unnecessarily.

14 C

15 You need to demonstrate your knowledge and understanding of the relevant material by clearly and logically considering a range of different aspects that are relevant to the context in the question, and show how these aspects interrelate.

Answers could include **any** from:

Suzie:
- has to do planning and marking in the evening; so will find it hard to make enough time
- has to bring home resources for planning and marking; this may be too much to carry if walking to and from school
- may become worried/anxious when she tries to exercise; because she feels her heart beating even faster/she is more out of breath
- may have good intentions for exercise after work; but she may prefer having a drink to relax and lose her motivation to exercise
- lives with her partner; who may support her to exercise more.

16 (a) (i) Actions could include any **three** from
- get more exercise
- eat a healthier diet
- stop taking drugs
- see a counsellor for depression
- take medication for depression.

(ii) Ways the actions could improve Chen's health and wellbeing could include any **three** from:
- Exercise releases endorphins, which will lift his mood.
- Exercise keeps his weight down so he will have better self-esteem/more chance of finding employment.
- Exercise will reduce his blood pressure/risk of heart disease/stroke/cancer.
- He will feel better about himself/fitter/mentally stronger if he is getting the nutrients he needs.
- Eating a healthier diet will reduce blood pressure/risk of heart disease/stroke/cancer.
- Stopping taking drugs will remove any anxiety caused by the drugs so may help reduce depression.
- He will not be as worried about money if he is not spending it on drugs.
- Counselling or medication will help reduce his depression.

16 (b) Answers could include any **two** from:
- Medication from the GP will help the depression and eventually lift Chen's mood; so he can take positive steps towards getting a new job.
- Attending support groups (face to face or online) will help Chen stop taking drugs, which will improve his physical health and emotional wellbeing.
- Chen's GP or a support group can give him information such as the Eatwell Guide/UK Physical Activity Guidelines, which will help him to eat a healthier diet/take more exercise.

17 (a) Answers could include any **two** from:

Geographical barrier:
- It is hard for Dave to get to appointments with his GP to get his medication as he is often travelling for his work.
- If he has to travel a long way on a particular day to meet a new client, he may be too far away to get back in time for an OT appointment.

Financial barrier:
- Dave can't afford to take time off work to attend appointments because he needs the money.

17 (b) Answers could include any **two** from:

Emotional/psychological obstacle:
- Dave may lack motivation; because if he has been going out drinking with clients, the alcohol may lessen his resolve to improve his diet/exercise.
- He may feel frustrated and give up; if he feels he is not making enough progress with his arm injury.

Time constraints:
- Dave works long hours during the week; which makes it difficult for him to attend gym classes/swimming regularly.

Unachievable targets:
- Dave has to eat out a lot; and the menu may not offer healthy options/he isn't able to cook healthy meals at home.

Lack of support:
- Dave is often away from home; so it isn't as easy for him to gain support from friends or family.

Lack of resources:
- Being away from home a lot; means that Dave does not have access to local fitness facilities, such as a leisure centre.

18 You need to demonstrate your knowledge and understanding of the relevant material by clearly and logically considering a range of different aspects that are relevant to the context in the question, and show how these aspects interrelate.

Answers could include **any** from:
- Mela may struggle with the emotionally addictive qualities of comfort eating, making it difficult to lose weight.
- Mela's increased weight might have lowered her self-esteem/made her embarrassed/reluctant to go out because of what others may think of her.
- Mela may be so conditioned to staying at home that she will find it hard to get motivated to go out to exercise/meet new people.
- Mela may be embarrassed to reach out to her few friends after habitually staying at home rather than socialising.
- Mela is likely to be grieving for her partner, which may make her feel too sad to go out.
- Mela may feel guilty about going out to try to enjoy herself when her partner has died.
- Mela may not have the confidence to go out on her own.
- As a bereaved partner, Mela may find it overwhelming or feel out of place when meeting other couples.
- Mela's age (56) may make it difficult to meet new people her own age, who likely have families, responsibilities and social circles of their own.

Practice assessment 2

(pages 11–20)

1 D

2 Answers could include any **two** from:
- reduced blood pressure
- reduced risk of heart attack/stroke/cancer/diabetes
- helps maintain a healthy weight/BMI
- better toned body/fitter/more flexible/stronger/more stamina
- better concentration/memory
- better sleep patterns
- less stressed/more relaxed/happier/better mood

- better self-esteem/personal satisfaction
- more endorphins in the body
- enjoy socialising with others while exercising.

3 Answers could include any **one** from:
- religion
- gender roles/expectations
- gender identity
- sexual orientation
- community participation.

4 B and E

5 Answers could include any **one** from:
- low self-esteem; due to feeling disliked and left out
- anxiety; due to worrying about being ignored in social situations
- stress; due to worrying about why they are being excluded
- increased blood pressure; resulting from the stress caused by being excluded
- insomnia/distress/anger/lack of concentration; due to worrying about being socially isolated
- turning to alcohol/smoking/substance abuse/self-harm; as a distraction from being socially isolated.

6 Answers could include any **two** from:
- less chance of accident/injury; as no trip hazards on the floor
- reduced chance of allergies/germs/infections; as germs/irritants are cleaned from surfaces
- feel happier; because surroundings look nice and are comfortable
- better able to concentrate on activities; because less distracted by unpleasant surroundings
- increased social interactions; as the inhabitants are happy to bring friends home.

7 Answers could include any **one** from:
- upset because in pain/feeling ill
- lonely because missing going out with friends/to school/college/university/work
- worried about the possible long-term effects
- concerned about the effects on family.

8 Answers could include any **two** from:
- make new friends; as they meet new people at work
- become more socially inclusive; as they meet people of different ages/from different cultures at work
- can socialise more; as can afford to go out/travel/take up new interests/go on courses with friends
- increased social skills; as they learn to work with people from other professions.

9 Answers could include any **one** from:
- no more periods/period pain
- reduced risk of pregnancy
- eventually no risk of pregnancy
- no need for hormonal birth control measures like the pill.

10 Answers could include any **two** from:
- upset; because they have less money to socialise with friends
- depressed; because they have less money for luxuries/to take up new interests/travel
- stressed/irritable/worried; because they have to look for another job
- low self-esteem; as they worry that they were made redundant because they are not good enough
- happy; because they have more time to spend with family and friends
- pleased; because they have more time to keep up with the news/learn new things on the internet
- excited; about the opportunity to find another job.

11 Low/below normal

12 Answers could include any **two** from:
- increased risk of high blood pressure/increased risk when under anaesthetic; because his heart is working harder to push blood round his larger body
- increased risk of heart attack/stroke at this time in his life; due to the extra weight he is carrying around
- joint problems; due to the extra weight causing more pressure on joints
- breathlessness; due to the extra weight restricting lung expansion
- becoming tired easily; due to his body systems being overworked.

13 A lack of exercise means the body is burning fewer calories. Muhammad therefore requires fewer calories to enter a caloric surplus, which results in weight gain and an increasing BMI.

14 B

15 You need to demonstrate your knowledge and understanding of the relevant material by clearly and logically considering a range of different aspects that are relevant to the context in the question, and show how these aspects interrelate.

Answers could include **any** from:

Muhammad:
- eats out to socialise with his wife and friends at weekends so may find it challenging to choose healthier options
- may find it easier to eat more healthily if his wife makes the same changes; they can agree to buy healthier food to have at home
- and his wife could invite friends to have dinner at their house, rather than go out to dinner, so that they cook healthier food and still socialise
- eats lunch out with his work colleagues, so he may find it hard to find/be motivated to pick healthy choices from the menu
- could pack a healthy lunch the night before to take to work, but he may miss relaxing with colleagues at lunchtime if they all go out
- may lack the time to go food shopping due to the demands of his job. Therefore enjoying, but also relying on, eating out at mealtimes rather than cooking healthy meals at home
- may not have major supermarkets in the local area, due to living in the countryside, and therefore finds it difficult to shop for healthier options
- could plan with colleagues to have one or two days per week where they all bring in a healthy lunch from home and eat together at work; giving Muhammad group accountability.

16 (a) (i) Actions could include any **three** from:
- get more exercise
- eat regularly by setting an alarm reminder on her phone
- eat a healthier diet
- get more sleep by stopping work several hours before bed or taking medication
- spend time outside.

   (ii) Ways the actions could improve Leanne's health and wellbeing could include any **three** from:
- Exercise releases endorphins, which will make Leanne feel happier/help her fall asleep/make her fitter with more stamina, strength and flexibility.
- Eating regularly will help increase Leanne's weight to the normal range.
- Eating a healthier diet will mean her body has the nutrients it needs to stay healthy/she will be mentally stronger if getting the nutrients she needs/will reduce Leanne's risk of developing osteoporosis/will strengthen her immune system.

- Getting more sleep will help her relax/concentrate better/be mentally stronger/help her body to repair.
- More exposure to fresh air and natural light could help to improve Leanne's circadian rhythm and therefore improve her sleep.

16 (b) Answers could include any **two** from:
- Leanne's friend/family can ring her at certain times to remind her to eat; to get her weight up to normal.
- Her husband can prepare her healthy snacks for during the day and/or call her for a healthy meal when he gets home from work; to make sure she eats healthily to get the nutrients her body and mind need to stay healthy.
- Her husband can remind her to stop working at a certain time and help her to relax by doing yoga/having a drink and a chat; to help her de-stress and improve her sleep.
- Her family/friend can take her out or exercise with her some evenings; so she can forget about work and relax before bed to help her get to sleep.

17 (a) Answers could include any **two** from:

Language barrier:
- The language barrier may make it harder for Abena to describe her symptoms/medical history to the medical staff; so it may take the medical staff longer to find out what is wrong and delay treatment.
- The language barrier may make it harder for the medical staff to find out her needs, wishes and circumstances; so she may not get the care she needs.
- Abena may be unable to ask the nursing staff to let her cousin know where she is, which may cause her anxiety and distress.

Resource barrier:
- The hospital may not have an interpreter available; so they can't explain what is wrong with her or find out key information which could help them treat her.
- Abena is in an isolation ward; so she will have less opportunity to communicate with the nurses about her illness.

Cultural barrier:
- The hospital may not be able to provide Abena with food that meets her dietary needs as they can't find out that information; so not eating may make her condition worse.

17 (b) Answers could include any **two** from:

Emotional/psychological obstacles:
- She may feel frightened and not want to go to her appointments; because she speaks little English/has had a bad experience already.
- She may not want to be a burden to her cousin by borrowing the bus fare.

Time constraints:
- The bus only runs twice a day so she has a long wait, which may mean she has to take a whole day for each appointment; which may make her not want to attend.

Lack of support:
- Abena may only know her cousin in the UK; which means she does not have a well-developed support network to help her get the care she needs.

18 You need to demonstrate your knowledge and understanding of the relevant material by clearly and logically considering a range of different aspects that are relevant to the context in the question, and show how these aspects interrelate.

Answers could include **any** from:
- James knows he will be different from the other students; so may be reluctant to start college.
- He may feel apprehensive about meeting lots of new young people and tutors/teachers; because they may not understand his communication needs at the beginning.
- As a result he may also feel socially isolated and find it harder to make friends.
- James may worry that he will fall behind if his interpreter cannot get in or the teaching staff don't speak clearly enough; because he may rely on reading lips.
- He will be aware that because of his medical condition, he has missed out on some of his learning; so he may be concerned that he will find himself unable to keep up with other students of the same age.
- However, he may feel happy and confident because his parents are very supportive; they have always done what they can to support him. For example, they may have made sure he learned sign language/to lip read, and that he caught up at home on any work missed when he was ill, so he didn't get behind.

Practice assessment 3

(pages 21–30)

1 D

2 Answers could include any **two** from:
- weight gain/obesity/increased BMI
- weight loss
- nutrient deficiency
- anaemia
- rickets
- poor growth
- tiredness
- depression
- increased blood pressure
- increased risk of heart disease/heart attack/stroke/cancer
- joint pain
- less flexible
- less stamina
- breathlessness
- tooth decay.

3 Answers could include any **one** from:
- employment
- unemployment
- income
- inheritance
- savings.

4 B and C

5 Answers could include any **one** of:
- social inclusion; as part of a group that worships together
- high self-esteem; as it feels good to belong to a group with the same beliefs
- lots of support; from people who share the same beliefs and values
- a positive attitude towards others; as all share the same values
- a sense of identity/belonging; as part of a community of people
- feeling supported/positive relationships; by/with people who value the same things.

6 Answers could include any **two** from:
- more chance of accident/overdose; because an individual is not in control of their actions when under the influence of a substance
- risk of addiction; which can put the individual in financial difficulties if they can't afford to feed their habit
- damage to organs and body systems; caused by the effects of

the substance on how the body functions, such as making the heart beat faster
- mood swings; due to the cravings for the substance and the effects of the substance on the brain
- unable to concentrate/distracted; due to effects of the substance, such as hallucinations
- social isolation as relationships worsen with family and friends; due to change in mood/attitude/asking for money/turning to crime to pay for the substance/poorer personal hygiene/ unacceptable behaviour when under the influence of the substance.

7 Answers could include any **one** from:
- feel closer to family and friends looking after you
- happy to spend more time with family
- more chance to talk and share feelings
- feel encouraged to reflect on life and find meaning through adversity.

8 Answers could include any **two** from:
- loss of strength/stamina; as they may lose their appetite
- may eat an unhealthy diet/put on weight; because they comfort eat and choose unhealthy foods
- may drink too much alcohol/turn to substance abuse; to try to ease the pain, leading to addiction/the negative health effects of a given substance
- tired and lacking in energy; due to the emotional turmoil
- loss of fitness; as no motivation to go out and exercise.

9 Answers could include any **one** from:
- unable to go out and socialise with friends
- unable to exercise with friends
- miss social opportunities with peers/colleagues at school, college, university or work
- miss opportunities to join social/community groups and make new friends
- may become socially isolated
- may experience discrimination due to the effects of the accident.

10 Answers could include any **two** from:
- unable to concentrate; because they are upset
- fewer learning opportunities (such as travel/courses to learn new skills); as they only have one income now/no partner to go with
- better able to focus and learn new things; as they are happier now they are not in an unsupportive relationship
- more learning opportunities; as they are driven to have a fresh start.

11 High/above normal

12 Answers could include any **two** from:
- Increased risk of heart attack/stroke; because the heart needs more oxygen than the body can provide.
- It could indicate high blood pressure; which means the heart is having to work too hard.
- Increased risk of collapse due to dizziness/breathlessness; so increased risk of injury.
- It could show that the heart isn't working properly; perhaps because of undiagnosed conditions, such as diabetes.

13 Answers could include any **one** from:
- Smoking/Nicotine raises blood pressure; causing the heart to already be beating faster so it takes longer to go down to normal.
- Smoking reduces lung capacity/increases the amount of carbon monoxide in the blood; so the heart needs to beat faster to pump enough oxygen around the body after exercise.
- Smoking scars the heart muscle, which means the heart beats

faster/less efficiently; so the heart takes longer to recover after exercise.

14 A

15 You need to demonstrate your knowledge and understanding of the relevant material by clearly and logically considering a range of different aspects that are relevant to the context in the question, and show how these aspects interrelate.

Answers could include **any** from:
Delphine:
- may be determined to cut down on smoking, but once she has had an alcoholic drink it reduces her motivation and she is likely to have a cigarette
- may have good intentions to stop smoking but will find it hard to say no when her friends are all going outside to smoke, which would leave her on her own
- will have cravings for the nicotine in cigarettes so will find it hard to give up
- will find it hard to stop smoking because she associates it with relaxing
- lives and works on her own, so will find it hard to stop smoking as she may have little support
- may find it easier to quit smoking because of the chest pains she is experiencing, which is a motivating factor for positive change.

16 (a) (i) Answers could include any **three** from:
- get more exercise
- eat a healthier diet by preparing a meal in advance
- cut down on or stop smoking
- reduce the amount of alcohol he drinks.

16 (a) (ii) Answers could include any **three** from:
- Exercise releases endorphins and improves fitness, which will make Eamonn get fitter/feel happier/ reduce his blood pressure/risk of heart disease/stroke/ cancer.
- A healthier diet will make Eamonn feel better about himself/lose weight/reduce his blood pressure/risk of heart disease/stroke/cancer.
- Cutting down on/stopping smoking will reduce breathlessness/risk of high blood pressure/lung cancer/emphysema/stroke/gum disease/asthma/ bronchitis/thrombosis.
- Reducing the amount of alcohol he drinks will reduce his risk of high blood pressure/weight gain/increased BMI/heart disease/stroke/cancer.

16 (b) Answers could include any **two** from:
- Eamonn could attend an online support group organised by a trained professional to help him give up smoking and drinking; which will offer him practical and emotional support by giving him praise and encouragement to keep trying.
- He could ask the practice nurse for information on aids to quit smoking, such as nicotine patches and gum; to give him a plan of action to stop smoking.
- He could make an appointment with a dietician to help him plan healthy meals; so he gets all the nutrients he needs for good health.
- He could consult a personal trainer; who can advise him how to fit exercise that is suitable for his age into his daily routine.

17 (a) Answers could include any **two** from:
Physical/geographical barrier:
- The hospital Rosie needs for her breathing exercises is a mile away up a steep hill; it may be hard for Rosie to walk up a steep hill with asthma.

Financial barriers:
- Rosie's dad earns the minimum wage and may not be able to afford the bus fare to the hospital; so they may have to walk, putting Rosie at risk of an asthma attack.
- Rosie's dad may not be able to afford to take time off work for Rosie's appointments; so Rosie may not get the help she needs.

Resources:
- There may not be the resources to fix the damp problem in the flat; so Rosie's asthma will continue to get worse.

17 (b)   Answers could include any **two** from:

Emotional/psychological:
- Rosie's dad is embarrassed to ask for help, such as help with the bus fare; so he may not always be able to take her to her appointments.
- Rosie's dad doesn't like to leave the flat; so doesn't always take her to her appointments.
- Rosie may feel anxious that the walk will make her asthma worse; so may not want to go to the hospital.

Time constraints:
- Rosie's regular appointment is on Friday afternoon; and Rosie's dad may not want Rosie to keep missing school.
- Her appointments for the breathing exercises and her visits to the practice nurse will be at different times; so even if they are on the same day, there will be time wasted waiting between appointments, meaning Rosie is missing school and her dad can't look for work.

Lack of support:
- Rosie's dad may not have anyone else that could take Rosie to the hospital; so she may end up missing important appointments.

18 You need to demonstrate your knowledge and understanding of the relevant material by clearly and logically considering a range of different aspects that are relevant to the context in the question, and show how these aspects interrelate.

Answers could include **any** from:
- Tahira can't stay behind after school for sports clubs or take part in sports activities at the weekend because she is looking after her mum; so her muscles and physical skills won't develop as fast as those of other children her age.
- Tahira will be getting some exercise and some fresh air during her PE lessons and breaks at school. She also does cleaning and other physical tasks in the home that other children may not be doing. These tasks are exercise that will help her physical development.
- She doesn't eat as well as she should as she and her mother eat only basic meals such as beans on toast; so she may not be getting all the nutrients she needs to grow and develop at the same rate as other children.
- She may not get outside at the weekends as much as some children; so she won't get much fresh air to clean lungs/ improve blood pressure/vitamin D from sunlight for healthy bone growth/muscle growth/immune system/heart.
- She has to get up early so may not get enough sleep. This may affect her growth, as during sleep growth hormones are released/sleep is important for healthy growth, repair and recovery.

Practice assessment 4

(pages 31–40)

1   A

2   Answers could include any **two** from:
- weight loss
- hair loss
- skin pallor
- tooth decay
- twitches
- withdrawal symptoms
- increased risk of accident/death
- increased risk of high blood pressure/heart disease/attack/ stroke/cancer
- increased risk of infection
- damage to organs
- addiction/cravings
- unable to concentrate/memory loss
- hallucinations
- sleep problems
- anxiety/depression/panic attacks/paranoia/aggression/low self-worth
- loss of friends/social isolation/breakdown of relationships
- loss of housing
- money/job problems
- risk of criminal record/imprisonment.

3   Answers could include any **one** from:
- inherited conditions
- physical ill health
- mental ill health
- physical abilities
- sensory impairments.

4   A and E

5   Answers could include **one** from:
- weight gain; as the body isn't getting the correct balance of nutrients/too many calories
- weight loss; as the body isn't getting the correct balance of nutrients/too few calories
- increased risk of diabetes; if too much sugar in the diet
- increased risk of osteoporosis or anaemia; if not enough calcium and vitamin D
- increased blood pressure; as heart has to work harder to pump blood round the body (or too much salt or fat in food)
- increased risk of high cholesterol; if eating too many fatty foods
- increased risk of heart disease/cancer/stroke; due to build-up of fats
- damage to joints/organs; due to carrying too much weight/fat.

6   Answers could include any **two** from:
- less risk of accidents; as have physical assistance if needed to do jobs in the home
- feel more contented/relaxed; as they have someone/people for company/to rely on/to do things with
- feel less anxious; as they have someone who will listen to them and help with their worries
- intellectual stimulation; due to having someone to talk/discuss things with
- social inclusion; as rarely alone/in regular contact with friends/ family
- higher self-esteem; due to unconditional love from family.

7   Answers could include any **one** from:
- may be unable to concentrate on anything else
- may lead to change of school/change of job so may need to learn new skills
- may neglect studies/any work done at home
- having to deal with legal documents/demands from solicitors can be intellectually demanding.

8 Answers could include any **two** from:
- excited to start college; because they are going to learn new things and make new friends
- relieved to be leaving school; as they are ready for a new challenge/fresh start
- increased self-esteem; as proud of how they have coped with change/can start to take care of themselves (cooking/managing own money)
- pride/increased self-esteem from feeling respected by family and friends; because of their achievement in getting into college.

9 Answers could include any **one** from:
- learning about home management
- learning financial management
- learning/developing/improving organisational skills
- able to concentrate on studies/work/new learning opportunities better.

10 Answers could include any **two** from:

The child will:
- develop gross motor skills; because they are taking part in activities such as new sports
- develop fine motor skills; such as being taught how to hold a pencil correctly/tie shoe laces/use a paintbrush
- get fitter/keep a healthy weight/increase flexibility; because of taking part in organised exercise
- get fresh air when playing; so keep lungs healthy
- eat a healthy lunch/snacks; through the school meals service
- stay hydrated; as they are encouraged to drink water during the day
- have less chance of accidents; as they are in a safe environment/taught how to stay physically safe
- have higher risk of accidents; because larger groups of children are playing together with the supervision of limited staff
- have higher risk of injury; due to the potential for physical bullying among groups of young children during social development
- have increased risk of illness; large numbers of children playing and studying together means that viruses spread quickly among peers.

11 Obese

12 Answers could include any **two** from:
- Possibly a greater risk of accident/injury; as low blood pressure can cause dizziness/fainting/blurred vision/nausea
- Katie may lack stamina/become over tired/have shallow breathing; as the body may not be getting enough oxygen.
- There is a risk of collapse as could go into shock and be cold/clammy/pale/shallow breathing/weak/rapid pulse; as the heart may not be working as well as it should.

13 Answers could include any **one** from:
- Her arteries will narrow due to a build-up of fat; so her heart has to work harder to push blood round her body, increasing her blood pressure.
- Her weight will increase due to too much bad cholesterol/fat/sugar; so putting more pressure on her heart.
- More fat in the body puts more pressure on organs such as kidneys; so they have to work harder which increases blood pressure.
- An unhealthy diet causes blood vessels to become stiffer so blood can't flow as easily; so the heart has to beat faster to push the blood through, increasing her blood pressure.

14 B

15 You need to demonstrate your knowledge and understanding of the relevant material by clearly and logically considering a

range of different aspects that are relevant to the context in the question, and show how these aspects interrelate.

Answers could include **any** from:
- Elliot regularly drinks alcohol to relax and when out with his husband and friends; so will find it hard to stop.
- He may be determined to cut down but once he has had one drink the alcohol will reduce his inhibitions; and he is likely to have more.
- He may find it easier to cut down the amount of alcohol he drinks if his husband tries to make the same changes; they can both agree to drink less and support each other.
- He can look for other ways to relax with his husband, such as doing yoga together; so that he has support in making positive changes.
- He can gradually reduce his working hours as he approaches retirement from his role as a magistrate; so he can concentrate on following a healthier lifestyle, including cutting back on alcohol.
- He could offer to be the designated driver when out in the evenings; so he is not tempted to drink alcohol.

16 (a) (i) Actions could include any **three** from:
- do low-impact exercise, such as swimming
- eat a healthier diet by cutting out/reducing the sweet foods
- increase the variety of vegetables, fruit, healthy grains and proteins in her diet
- change from sugary drinks to low-sugar diet drinks, herbal teas or water.

(ii) Ways the actions could improve Priya's health and wellbeing could include any **three** from:
- exercise releases endorphins, which will make Priya feel happier
- exercise will help her to stop putting weight on/reduce blood pressure/risk of heart disease/stroke/cancer
- eating a healthier diet will make Priya feel better about herself/fitter/lose weight/ reduce blood pressure/risk of heart disease/stroke/cancer
- eating a more varied diet will help Priya get all the nutrients she needs to aid her recovery
- cutting out sugary drinks will reduce the number of calories she is consuming; so she will lose weight/be better hydrated/reduce her risk of developing diabetes.

16 (b) Answers could include any **two** from:
- Priya's parents can stop buying sweet items or replace them with low-sugar alternatives; so she isn't tempted.
- Her family can also eat healthily; so that she has moral support.
- Her parents can buy low-sugar drinks, such as bottled water, herbal teas and fruit to flavour water; so she gets used to drinking those instead of sugary drinks.
- Her younger brother could offer to go swimming with her; to help her stick to her exercise plans.

17 (a) Answers could include any **two** from:

Access to resources:
- The hospital that Ivan has to attend is 5 miles away; so it will be difficult for him to get there as he can't drive for 12 months.

Geographical barriers:
- Ivan's GP's surgery is 3 miles away in a different direction; so Ivan will have to travel by bus or taxi; which is expensive so he may miss appointments if he cannot afford the fare.
- The hospital is not local to him; so it will take a long time for him to get there, which could mean he misses appointments.

17 (b)   Answers could include any **two** from:

Emotional/psychological:
- Ivan may be worried about the doctor's reaction if they find out he has been drinking against medical advice; so he may not be honest, which could put his health at risk.
- He is worried about his tumour returning/having a seizure; so he may miss appointments to avoid hearing bad news.
- He may also be worried about the stigma of going to the doctor's to discuss his feelings of anxiety/social withdrawal.

Time constraints:
- It takes a long time to get to appointments as they are so far away; so he may not be able to go.

Lack of support:
- He hasn't been in touch his friends much; so he may feel that he can't ask them for help such as a lift to an appointment.

18   You need to demonstrate your knowledge and understanding of the relevant material by clearly and logically considering a range of different aspects that are relevant to the context in the question, and show how these aspects interrelate.

Answers could include **any** from:
- Noah receives no help from his mum with his reading or anything else that will help him learn at home; so he isn't intellectually stimulated/is likely to fall behind those children who do get such support.
- Noah sometimes misses school because his mother doesn't take him; so he will fall behind his classmates.
- By missing school, Noah is missing out on intellectual development that is gained through social interactions/ conversations with his peers.
- By missing school, Noah is missing out on physical exercise at breaks and during PE, as both fresh air and learning new skills/ rules help intellectual development.
- Noah's dad often comes home when Noah is getting ready for bed so it is unlikely that he will read Noah a bedtime story; so a chance is missed to discuss each page of a book to help his intellectual development.
- Because Noah's mum is usually on the phone and he only sees his dad at bedtime, he is not included in any adult conversation; so he is missing the chance to extend his vocabulary/increase his knowledge and understanding of the world.
- Because Noah is not encouraged to do anything related to school, he will think it is normal not to do any learning at home; so he will grow up not knowing that learning also takes place outside school.
- Because Noah's mum thinks he should miss school due to minor issues such as the weather, Noah may develop the belief that it is normal to give up in the face of minor challenges.

Notes

Notes

Notes

Notes